Vital Nutrients Unveiled

for Essential Vitamins and

Minerals in the Body

The Ultimate Guide to Vitamin D, Vitamin C, and Iodine for Optimal Health and Wellness.

By Dr. Cynthia C. Fenton.

Table of content

Introduction

In our quest for a healthy and vibrant life, we often come across various nutrients that are believed to hold the key to our well-being. Among these, Vitamin D, Vitamin C, and Iodine stand out as crucial players in supporting our overall health. These essential nutrients play diverse roles in our bodies, influencing everything from bone health to immune function and brain development.

Vitamin D, often referred to as the "sunshine vitamin," has gained considerable attention in recent years. It is unique because our bodies can produce it when our skin is exposed to sunlight. Additionally, Vitamin D can also be obtained from certain food sources and supplements. This essential nutrient plays a pivotal role in the absorption of calcium and phosphorus, promoting strong bones and teeth. Furthermore, Vitamin D is known to contribute to immune system regulation and mental well-being. It has been linked to a reduced risk of chronic diseases, including certain types of cancer, cardiovascular disease, and autoimmune disorders.

Similarly, Vitamin C, also known as ascorbic acid, has long been recognized for its powerful antioxidant properties. It is found abundantly in fruits and vegetables, particularly citrus fruits, berries, and leafy greens. Vitamin C plays a vital role in collagen synthesis, a protein that provides structure to our skin, bones, and blood vessels. It also enhances iron absorption, supports immune function, and helps protect cells from oxidative stress. Furthermore, Vitamin C contributes to the maintenance of healthy gums and aids in wound healing. Its immune-boosting effects have gained particular attention, making it a popular nutrient during times of increased susceptibility to illnesses.

Moving on to Iodine, a trace mineral often overlooked but no less important, it plays a critical role in the production of thyroid hormones. The thyroid gland, located in the neck, is responsible for regulating metabolism, growth, and development. Iodine deficiency can lead to various health issues, including goiter (enlarged thyroid gland), hypothyroidism (underactive thyroid), and cognitive impairments. Ensuring an adequate intake of iodine is essential for maintaining thyroid health, supporting normal growth and development, and optimizing metabolic processes in the body.

The importance of these three nutrients extends beyond their individual roles. They also interact synergistically, complementing each other's functions to promote overall health and well-being. For instance, Vitamin D aids in calcium absorption, while Vitamin C enhances iron absorption. Moreover, all three nutrients contribute to the immune systems optimal functioning, safeguarding our bodies against pathogens and reducing the risk of infections.

Understanding the sources and recommended daily intakes of these nutrients is vital for incorporating them into our diets. While sunlight exposure is a natural source of Vitamin D, food sources like fatty fish, fortified dairy products, and certain mushrooms can also provide this nutrient. Vitamin C-rich foods encompass a wide range of fruits and vegetables, including oranges, strawberries, bell peppers, and broccoli. Iodine can be obtained from iodized salt, seafood, dairy products, and seaweed.

In situations where dietary intake may be insufficient or specific health conditions warrant it, supplementation can be considered.

Chapter one

Overview of Essential Nutrients

Nutrition forms the foundation of our well-being, providing the essential building blocks for growth, repair, and maintenance of our bodies. Essential nutrients play a fundamental role in this process, ensuring that our bodies function optimally. In this section, we will delve into the diverse categories of essential nutrients, exploring their importance and the functions they serve in the human body.

Macronutrients:

Macronutrients are nutrients required in relatively large amounts and provide the bulk of our daily energy needs. They include carbohydrates, proteins, and fats.

Carbohydrate: Simple carbohydrates, like those found in sugar and honey, provide quick energy, while complex carbohydrates, found in whole grains and starchy vegetables, provide sustained energy and valuable dietary fiber.

Proteins: Proteins are essential for the growth, repair, and maintenance of body tissues. Dietary sources of proteins include meat, fish, poultry, dairy products, legumes, and plant-based sources such as soy and quinoa. Proteins also play a crucial role in enzyme production, immune function, and hormone synthesis.

Fats: Fats are a concentrated source of energy and serve as a storage form for energy in the body. Healthy fats, such as those found in avocados, nuts, seeds, and olive oil, are essential for overall health. However, it's important to limit the intake of unhealthy saturated and Tran's fats found in fried foods and processed snacks.

Micronutrients:

Micronutrients are essential in smaller quantities but are equally vital for our health. They include vitamins and minerals.

Vitamins: They can be classified into two categories: fat-soluble vitamins (A, D, E, and K) and water-soluble vitamins (B vitamins and vitamin C). Each vitamin has specific roles in maintaining health, ranging from supporting the immune system (vitamin C) to promoting healthy vision (vitamin A).

Minerals: They include macro minerals like calcium, phosphorus, magnesium, sodium, and potassium, as well as trace minerals like iron, zinc, copper, iodine, and selenium. Minerals contribute to bone health, nerve function, muscle contraction, and fluid balance. Food sources rich in minerals include dairy products, seafood, leafy greens, nuts, and seeds.

Water: Water is often overlooked as a nutrient, but it is crucial for our survival. It is involved in nearly every bodily function, including digestion, circulation, temperature regulation, and waste removal. Staying adequately hydrated is essential for optimal physical and mental performance.

Phytonutrients: Phytonutrients are natural compounds found in plant-based foods that offer numerous health benefits. They include antioxidants, flavonoids, carotenoids, and other plant compounds. Phytonutrients contribute to reducing inflammation, boosting the immune system, and protecting against chronic diseases like cancer and heart disease. Colorful fruits, vegetables, herbs, and spices are excellent sources of phytonutrients.

Understanding the importance of these essential nutrients and incorporating a well-balanced diet that includes a variety of nutrient-rich foods is vital for overall health and well-being. Each nutrient has its unique role in supporting bodily functions, and deficiencies or imbalances can lead to health issues. It is crucial to consult with healthcare professionals or registered dietitians to ensure that dietary needs are met and to address any specific nutrient requirements or concerns.

Importance of Vitamin D, Vitamin C, and Iodine

Vitamin D, Vitamin C, and Iodine are three essential nutrients that play crucial roles in maintaining our health and well-being. Each nutrient brings a unique set of benefits and functions to the table, contributing to various bodily processes and promoting optimal physiological function. In this section, we will explore the importance of

Vitamin D, Vitamin C, and Iodine in detail, shedding light on their significant impact on human health.

Importance of Vitamin D

Vitamin D, often referred to as the "sunshine vitamin," is unique among vitamins because our bodies can synthesize it when our skin is exposed to sunlight. Additionally, it can also be obtained from certain food sources and supplements. The importance of Vitamin D goes far beyond its role in calcium absorption and bone health.

Bone Health and Calcium Regulation:

Vitamin D plays a critical role in maintaining bone health by promoting calcium absorption in the intestines and reducing calcium loss in the kidneys. It ensures that there is an adequate supply of calcium and phosphorus in the body, which are essential for building and maintaining strong bones and teeth. Insufficient Vitamin D levels can lead to weakened bones, increased risk of fractures, and conditions like rickets in children and osteomalacia in adults.

Immune Function:

Vitamin D is involved in modulating the immune system, enhancing its ability to fight against infections and promoting overall immune health. It helps activate immune cells, such as T cells and macrophages that are crucial for recognizing and destroying pathogens. Adequate Vitamin D levels have been associated with reduced risk of respiratory infections, autoimmune diseases, and certain cancers.

Mental Well-being:

Vitamin D receptors are found in areas of the brain associated with mood regulation, and adequate levels of Vitamin D may help support healthy brain function and emotional well-being.

Cardiovascular Health:

Vitamin D has been shown to play a role in cardiovascular health. It may help regulate blood pressure, reduce inflammation, and improve blood vessel function. Some studies have indicated a potential association between Vitamin D deficiency and an increased risk of cardiovascular diseases such as hypertension, heart disease, and stroke.

Cancer Prevention:

There is growing evidence suggesting that Vitamin D may play a role in reducing the risk of certain types of cancers, including colorectal, breast, prostate, and pancreatic cancers. Vitamin D has been shown to inhibit cell proliferation, promote cell differentiation, and modulate apoptosis (programmed cell death) in cancer cells.

Autoimmune Disorders:

Vitamin D may have a modulatory effect on the immune system, making it an area of interest in the field of autoimmune diseases. Studies have suggested that Vitamin D deficiency may contribute to an increased risk of autoimmune conditions such as multiple sclerosis, rheumatoid arthritis, and type 1 diabetes.

Potential Interactions and Synergistic Effects:

Vitamin D interacts with various biological pathways and may have synergistic effects with other nutrients. For example, Vitamin D and calcium work together to support bone health, and Vitamin D and Vitamin K may have a synergistic role in cardiovascular health. Understanding these interactions can help optimize health outcomes.

Importance of Vitamin C:

It is renowned for its potent antioxidant properties and plays numerous vital roles in maintaining overall health.

Antioxidant Protection:

Vitamin C acts as a powerful antioxidant, neutralizing harmful free radicals and protecting cells from oxidative damage. This antioxidant activity helps prevent cellular aging, reduces inflammation, and may contribute to a decreased risk of chronic diseases such as heart disease, certain cancers, and neurodegenerative disorders.

Immune System Support:

It enhances the production and function of immune cells, such as white blood cells and antibodies, helping the body fight against infections and diseases. It also supports the function of the skin, which serves as a physical barrier against pathogens.

Collagen Synthesis:

Collagen is a protein that provides structure and strength to our skin, bones, joints, and other connective tissues. Vitamin C plays a key role in the production of collagen, which is essential for wound healing, tissue repair, and maintaining the health and elasticity of the skin. It also supports the health of blood vessels, cartilage, and gums.

Iron Absorption:

By reducing iron to its more absorbable form, Vitamin C helps combat iron deficiency anemia, a common nutritional deficiency. Including sources of Vitamin C with iron-rich foods can significantly improve iron absorption and prevent iron deficiency.

Chapter two

Vitamin D

Vitamin D, often referred to as the "sunshine vitamin," is a unique and essential nutrient that plays a crucial role in supporting overall health and well-being. From its importance in bone health to its involvement in immune function and beyond, Vitamin D offers a multitude of benefits that are vital for maintaining optimal physiological function. In this section, we will delve into the essentials of Vitamin D, exploring its sources, functions, recommended intakes, deficiency risks, and supplementation considerations.

Sources of Vitamin D

When ultraviolet B (UVB) rays from the sun interact with the skin, a chemical reaction occurs, converting a cholesterol compound into a precursor form of Vitamin D3. This inactive form is further processed by the liver and kidneys, eventually converting it into the active form of Vitamin D known as calcitriol.

While sunlight is the most efficient source of Vitamin D, certain dietary sources can provide this essential nutrient as well. These include:

1. Fatty Fish:

Fatty fish like salmon, mackerel, sardines, and trout are excellent sources of Vitamin D. They contain high levels of this nutrient, particularly when wild-caught or exposed to natural sunlight. Regular consumption of fatty fish can contribute significantly to Vitamin D intake.

2. Fortified Foods:

Due to the recognition of the prevalence of Vitamin D deficiency in some populations, certain food products, such as dairy products (milk, yogurt, and cheese), orange juice, and breakfast cereals, are often fortified with Vitamin D. Fortified foods can provide a convenient dietary source of this essential nutrient, especially for individuals with limited sunlight exposure or those with specific dietary restrictions.

3. Eggs:

Egg yolks contain small amounts of Vitamin D, making them a modest source of this nutrient. However, it's important to note that the Vitamin D content in eggs can vary depending on the diet of the chickens.

4. Mushrooms:

Some varieties of mushrooms have the ability to produce Vitamin D2 when exposed to ultraviolet light. These include shiitake, maitake, and morel mushrooms. However, the Vitamin D content in mushrooms can be highly variable and is dependent on their growing conditions.

Functions and Benefits of Vitamin D

Vitamin D serves a wide range of functions in the body, extending beyond its well-known role in bone health. Some of the essential functions and benefits of Vitamin D include:

- **Calcium and Phosphorus Absorption:**

Vitamin D plays a vital role in the absorption of calcium and phosphorus from the intestines. It helps regulate calcium levels in the blood, ensuring an adequate supply for the development and maintenance of strong bones and teeth. Without sufficient Vitamin D, the body may struggle to absorb these essential minerals, leading to weakened bones and an increased risk of conditions such as rickets in children and osteomalacia in adults.

- **Bone Health:**

Vitamin D works in synergy with calcium to maintain optimal bone health. It promotes the mineralization of bones and helps regulate the balance between bone formation and resumption. Adequate Vitamin D levels are essential for maintaining bone density, reducing the risk of fractures and osteoporosis, and supporting skeletal integrity.

- **Muscle Function:**

Vitamin D plays a role in muscle function and strength. Adequate Vitamin D levels may contribute to improved muscle performance, balance, and reduced risk of falls in older adults.

- **Immune System Support:**

It modulates the immune response and helps defend against pathogens. It enhances the production and activity of immune cells, such as T cells and macrophages, and promotes an appropriate inflammatory response. Adequate Vitamin D levels have been associated with a reduced risk of respiratory infections, autoimmune diseases, and certain cancers.

- **Mental Well-being:**

Emerging research suggests a connection between Vitamin D and mental health. Adequate Vitamin D levels may contribute to maintaining positive mental well-being.

Cardiovascular Health:

Vitamin D may play a role in cardiovascular health. It has been associated with a reduced risk of hypertension, heart disease, and stroke. Vitamin D may help regulate blood pressure, reduce inflammation, improve blood vessel function, and influence other factors related to cardiovascular health.

Recommended Daily Intake of Vitamin D

The recommended daily intake of Vitamin D can vary depending on factors such as age, sex, health status, and geographical location. 3.1 Infants and Children:

Infants up to 12 months of age require 400-1,000 international units (IU) of Vitamin D per day, either from breast milk, infant formula, or supplementation. Children aged 1-18 years require 600-1,000 IU per day.

Adults:

Adults aged 19-70 years require 600-800 IU of Vitamin D per day. However, individuals with limited sunlight exposure, dark skin pigmentation, or specific health conditions may require higher doses. Older adults above the age of 70 may benefit from higher Vitamin D intakes (800-1,000 IU per day) to support bone health and muscle function.

Supplementation Considerations:

Vitamin D supplementation may be necessary for individuals with limited sunlight exposure, those with darker skin pigmentation, or those at higher risk of deficiency. Individuals with specific health conditions or those taking certain medications should consult healthcare professionals to 3.1 Infants and Children:

Infants up to 12 months of age require 400-1,000 international units (IU) of Vitamin D per day, either from breast milk, infant formula, or supplementation. Children aged 1-18 years require 600-1,000 IU per day.

Deficiency Risks and Health Implications

Vitamin D deficiency is a global health concern, affecting various populations across different age groups. Factors contributing to Vitamin D deficiency include limited sunlight exposure, inadequate dietary intake, dark skin pigmentation, geographic location, cultural practices, and certain medical conditions.

- Rickets and Osteomalacia:

Severe Vitamin D deficiency during childhood can lead to rickets, a condition characterized by impaired bone growth, weak and soft bones, skeletal deformities, and increased fracture risk. In adults, Vitamin D deficiency can cause osteomalacia, a condition where the bones become weak, brittle, and more prone to fractures.

- Increased Risk of Falls and Fractures:

Inadequate Vitamin D levels can increase the risk of falls and fractures, particularly in older adults. Vitamin D plays a crucial role in muscle function and balance, and deficiency can contribute to muscle weakness, impaired coordination, and reduced bone density.

- Impaired Immune Function:

Vitamin D deficiency has been associated with compromised immune function and an increased susceptibility to infections. Insufficient Vitamin D levels may impair the body's ability to mount an effective immune response, leading to an increased risk of respiratory infections, autoimmune diseases, and other infectious diseases.

- Cardiovascular Risks:

Some studies have suggested an association between Vitamin D deficiency and an increased risk of cardiovascular diseases, including hypertension, heart disease, and stroke. Vitamin D plays a role in regulating blood pressure, reducing inflammation, and improving blood vessel function. Insufficient levels may contribute to cardiovascular risks.

- Mental Health Disorders:

Low Vitamin D levels have been linked to an increased risk of mood disorders, such as depression and seasonal affective disorder (SAD).

Supplementation Considerations and Safety

Vitamin D supplementation may be necessary in cases of deficiency or when recommended intakes cannot be met through sunlight exposure and dietary sources alone. Supplementation should be done under the guidance of healthcare professionals, who can assess individual needs and determine appropriate dosages.

It is important to note that excessive intake of Vitamin D can lead to toxicity, causing symptoms such as nausea, vomiting, poor appetite, excessive thirst, frequent urination, and, in severe cases, kidney damage. The tolerable upper intake level (UL) for Vitamin D in adults is set at 4,000 IU per day. However, it is advisable to consult healthcare professionals to determine individual requirements and to monitor blood levels to ensure optimal and safe intake.

Functions and Benefits of Vitamin D

Key functions and benefits of Vitamin D in detail:

Calcium and Phosphorus Absorption:

Vitamin D plays a fundamental role in the absorption of calcium and phosphorus from the intestines. It helps regulate the levels of these minerals in the blood, ensuring an adequate supply for the development and maintenance of strong bones and teeth. Without sufficient Vitamin D, the body may struggle to absorb these essential minerals, leading to weakened bones and an increased risk of conditions such as rickets in children and osteomalacia in adults.

Bone Health and Density:

Vitamin D works synergistically with calcium to maintain optimal bone health. It promotes the mineralization of bones and helps regulate the balance between bone formation and resumption. Adequate Vitamin D levels are essential for maintaining bone density, reducing the risk of fractures and osteoporosis, and supporting skeletal integrity throughout life.

Muscle Function and Strength:

Vitamin D plays a role in muscle function, strength, and coordination. It helps regulate the contraction and relaxation of muscles by influencing the uptake and utilization of calcium within muscle cells. Adequate Vitamin D levels may contribute to improved muscle performance, balance, and reduced risk of falls, particularly in older adults.

Immune System Support:

It plays a regulatory role in immune function, helping to modulate the immune response and defend against pathogens. Vitamin D enhances the production and activity of immune cells, such as T cells and macrophages, which are key players in the immune defense against infections and diseases. Adequate Vitamin D levels have been associated with a reduced risk of respiratory infections, autoimmune diseases, and certain cancers.

Anti-inflammatory Effects:

Vitamin D exhibits anti-inflammatory properties. It helps regulate the body's inflammatory response, reducing excessive inflammation that can contribute to chronic diseases such as cardiovascular disease, diabetes, and autoimmune disorders. By modulating inflammation, Vitamin D may help maintain a balanced immune system and promote overall health.

Mood Regulation and Mental Well-being:

Emerging research suggests a link between Vitamin D and mental health. Adequate Vitamin D levels may contribute to maintaining positive mental well-being and supporting cognitive function.

Cardiovascular Health:

Vitamin D may play a role in cardiovascular health. It has been associated with a reduced risk of hypertension (high blood pressure), heart disease, and stroke. Vitamin D may help regulate blood pressure, reduce inflammation, improve blood vessel function, and influence other factors related to cardiovascular health.

Regulation of Gene Expression:

Vitamin D acts as a hormone in the body, influencing the expression of numerous genes involved in various physiological processes. It has been shown to affect gene regulation related to cell growth, differentiation, apoptosis, and immune function. By modulating gene expression, Vitamin D can have far-reaching effects on overall health and well-being.

Overall Health and Disease Prevention:

Adequate Vitamin D levels have been associated with a reduced risk of several chronic diseases, including cardiovascular disease, diabetes, multiple sclerosis, rheumatoid arthritis, and certain types of cancer. By supporting optimal physiological function, Vitamin D contributes to overall health and plays a crucial role in disease prevention.

To ensure sufficient Vitamin D levels, it is recommended to obtain sensible sun exposure, consume Vitamin D-rich foods (such as fatty fish and fortified dairy products), and consider supplementation when necessary, under the guidance of healthcare professionals. Regular monitoring of Vitamin D levels through blood tests can help determine individual requirements and optimize intake for optimal health and well-being.

Blood Testing and Individual Assessment:

To determine an individual's Vitamin D status and needs, healthcare professionals may recommend blood testing to measure the levels of 25-hydroxyvitamin D [25(OH)D], the primary circulating form of Vitamin D. Based on the results, personalized recommendations can be made to address deficiencies or optimize Vitamin D levels.

Balancing Sun Exposure and Dietary Sources:

Achieving optimal Vitamin D levels involves striking a balance between sensible sun exposure and dietary intake. Sensible sun exposure, without excessive sunburn risk, allows the body to naturally produce Vitamin D.

Deficiency Symptoms and Health Risks

Vitamin D deficiency is a global health concern, affecting various populations across different age groups and geographic locations. Inadequate Vitamin D levels can have significant health implications and increase the risk of various conditions. Let's explore the symptoms and health risks associated with Vitamin D deficiency:

Bone Health Impairment:

Inadequate Vitamin D levels can lead to impaired bone mineralization, weakening the bones and increasing the risk of conditions such as rickets in children and osteomalacia in adults. Symptoms may include bone pain, muscle weakness, fractures, and skeletal deformities in severe cases.

Increased Risk of Osteoporosis:

Vitamin D deficiency can contribute to reduced bone density and an increased risk of osteoporosis, a condition characterized by fragile bones. Osteoporosis can make individuals more susceptible to fractures, particularly in the spine, hips, and wrists.

Muscle Weakness and Balance Issues:

Vitamin D plays a role in muscle function and strength. Inadequate levels can contribute to muscle weakness, fatigue, and impaired balance, increasing the risk of falls and fractures, especially in older adults.

Increased Susceptibility to Infections:

Deficiency can compromise immune function, leading to an increased susceptibility to infections. Respiratory tract infections, such as the common cold, influenza, and pneumonia, are particularly associated with low Vitamin D levels.

Mood Disorders:

Emerging evidence suggests a link between Vitamin D deficiency and mood disorders such as depression and seasonal affective disorder (SAD). Low Vitamin D levels have been associated with an increased risk of depressive symptoms and poor mental well-being.

Cardiovascular Risks:

Vitamin D deficiency has been associated with an increased risk of cardiovascular diseases, including hypertension (high blood pressure), heart disease, and stroke. Inadequate Vitamin D levels may contribute to elevated blood pressure, inflammation, and impaired blood vessel function.

Autoimmune Conditions:

Vitamin D plays a regulatory role in immune function and has been implicated in autoimmune diseases such as multiple sclerosis, rheumatoid arthritis, and type 1 diabetes. Deficiency may contribute to an increased risk of developing or exacerbating these conditions.

Cancer Susceptibility:

Some studies have suggested a potential association between Vitamin D deficiencies and an increased risk of certain types of cancer, including colon, breast, prostate, and pancreatic cancers. Adequate Vitamin D levels may help regulate cell growth, inhibit the proliferation of cancer cells, and promote programmed cell death (apoptosis).

Vitamin D Supplements

Vitamin D supplementation can be an effective strategy to ensure adequate intake, especially in individuals with limited sun exposure, those at higher risk of deficiency, or when recommended daily intakes cannot be met through natural sources alone. Let's explore the key considerations and benefits of Vitamin D supplementation:

Types of Vitamin D Supplements:

Vitamin D supplements are available in various forms, including capsules, tablets, soft gels, and liquid drops. The most common forms of Vitamin D used in supplements are Vitamin D2 (ergocalciferol) and Vitamin D3 (cholecalciferol). Vitamin D3, which is the same form synthesized in the skin in response to sunlight, is considered more bioavailable and preferred for supplementation.

Determining Supplement Dosage:

The appropriate dosage of Vitamin D supplementation depends on individual factors, including age, health status, existing deficiencies, and specific needs. Healthcare professionals or registered dietitians can assess individual requirements and recommend the most suitable dosage. General guidelines for Vitamin D supplementation include:

Infants: Supplementation with Vitamin D is often recommended for breastfed infants, with a typical dosage ranging from 400 to 1,000 IU per day, depending on the infant's age and specific needs.

Children and Adults: For children and adults, typical dosage ranges from 600 to 2,000 IU per day, depending on age, risk factors, and specific requirements. Higher doses may be prescribed for individuals with known deficiencies or those at higher risk of deficiency.

Older Adults: Older adults, particularly those above the age of 70, may benefit from higher Vitamin D supplementation doses ranging from 800 to 2,000 IU per day to support bone health and muscle function.

Combined Formulations:

Vitamin D supplements are often combined with other nutrients, such as calcium or magnesium, to support bone health and mineral balance. These combination supplements can provide a convenient way to address multiple nutrient needs simultaneously. However, it's important to ensure that the combined dosage aligns with individual requirements and that calcium and Vitamin D ratios are appropriate.

Timing and Duration:

The timing and duration of Vitamin D supplementation may vary based on individual needs and healthcare professional recommendations. Some individuals may require continuous supplementation, while others may benefit from periodic or seasonal supplementation. Regular monitoring of Vitamin D levels through blood tests can help assess efficacy and guide adjustments in supplementation strategies.

Potential Interactions and Precautions:

While Vitamin D supplementation is generally considered safe, it's important to be aware of potential interactions with certain medications. Some medications, such as corticosteroids, anticonvulsants, and certain weight loss drugs, can affect Vitamin D metabolism and absorption. Individuals taking these medications should consult healthcare professionals to determine appropriate supplementation strategies.

Adverse Effects and Toxicity:

Vitamin D toxicity is rare but can occur with excessive intake of supplements. The tolerable upper intake level (UL) for Vitamin D in adults is set at 4,000 IU per day. Intake above this threshold can lead to symptoms such as nausea, vomiting, poor appetite, excessive thirst, frequent urination, and, in severe cases, kidney damage. It's important to follow healthcare professional recommendations and avoid self-prescribing high-dose Vitamin D supplements.

Personalized Guidance:

Vitamin D supplementation should be done under the guidance of healthcare professionals or registered dietitians. They can assess individual needs, consider existing health conditions and medications, and provide personalized recommendations on dosage, duration, and appropriate supplementation strategies.

Chapter three

Vitamin C

Vitamin C, also known as ascorbic acid, is a water-soluble vitamin that plays a critical role in maintaining overall health and well-being. It is considered an essential nutrient as the human body cannot produce it on its own, and therefore, it must be obtained through dietary sources or supplements.

Vitamin C is renowned for its powerful antioxidant properties, which help protect the body against the harmful effects of free radicals – unstable molecules that can damage cells and contribute to various health conditions. As an antioxidant, Vitamin C helps neutralize these free radicals, reducing oxidative stress and promoting cellular health.

Beyond its antioxidant role, Vitamin C is involved in numerous important bodily functions. It plays a vital role in collagen synthesis, a protein crucial for the health of connective tissues, skin, blood vessels, and cartilage. This vitamin also supports immune function by enhancing the activity of immune cells and promoting the production of antibodies.

Understanding Vitamin C

Vitamin C, also known as ascorbic acid, is a water-soluble vitamin that holds significant importance for our overall health and well-being. Let's delve into the key aspects of this essential nutrient to gain a comprehensive understanding:

Chemical Properties:

Vitamin C is a powerful antioxidant, meaning it has the ability to neutralize harmful free radicals in the body. As a water-soluble vitamin, it dissolves in water and is not stored in the body for extended periods. This highlights the importance of regular intake through dietary sources or supplements.

Health Benefits:

It plays a vital role in collagen synthesis, promoting healthy skin, blood vessels, cartilage, and connective tissues. Additionally, it aids in wound healing, supports immune function by enhancing the activity of immune cells, and contributes to the production of antibodies.

Antioxidant Properties:

One of the most notable features of Vitamin C is its potent antioxidant properties. Antioxidants protect the body against oxidative stress caused by free radicals, which can damage cells and contribute to various diseases. By neutralizing these free radicals, Vitamin C helps reduce the risk of chronic conditions such as heart disease, certain cancers, and neurodegenerative disorders.

Dietary Sources:

While Vitamin C cannot be produced by the body, it can be obtained through dietary sources. Common food sources rich in Vitamin C include citrus fruits (such as oranges and grapefruits), berries (like strawberries and blueberries), kiwi fruit, papaya, pineapple, bell peppers, broccoli, and leafy green vegetables. Consuming a varied diet with these nutrient-rich foods can help ensure adequate Vitamin C intake.

Recommended Daily Intake:

For most adults, the recommended dietary allowance (RDA) is around 75-90 milligrams per day for women and 90 milligrams per day for men. However, certain conditions or situations, such as pregnancy, lactation, smoking, or illness, may warrant higher intakes, and healthcare professionals can provide specific guidance.

Supplementation:

While a well-balanced diet can generally meet the Vitamin C needs of most individuals, certain circumstances may call for supplementation. This includes individuals with limited dietary intake, malabsorption issues, or those who have specific health conditions requiring higher Vitamin C levels. Supplements are available in various forms, such as tablets, capsules, powders, and effervescent tablets, and should be used under healthcare professional guidance.

Safety and Precautions:

Vitamin C is considered safe for most individuals when consumed within the recommended daily limits. However, extremely high doses from supplementation may lead to gastrointestinal discomfort, diarrhea, or, in rare cases, kidney stones. It's important to follow healthcare professional recommendations and avoid excessive supplementation.

Roles and Benefits of Vitamin C

Vitamin C, also known as ascorbic acid, serves diverse roles in the body and offers numerous benefits for overall health and well-being. Let's explore the key roles and benefits of Vitamin C in detail:

Antioxidant Protection:

It scavenges these free radicals, neutralizing their harmful effects and reducing oxidative stress. By combating oxidative stress, Vitamin C contributes to the prevention of chronic diseases, such as cardiovascular diseases, certain cancers, and neurodegenerative disorders.

Collagen Synthesis:

Vitamin C plays a crucial role in the synthesis of collagen, a protein found in connective tissues, skin, blood vessels, and bones. Collagen provides structural support and helps maintain the integrity and elasticity of these tissues. Adequate Vitamin C levels are essential for proper collagen formation, promoting healthy skin, wound healing, and maintaining the health of blood vessels and bones.

Immune Function:

Vitamin C plays an integral role in supporting immune function. It enhances the activity of immune cells, including white blood cells, and promotes the production of antibodies. Vitamin C also helps stimulate the production of certain immune cells, enhancing their ability to combat infections. Adequate Vitamin C intake is essential for a robust immune response and reducing the risk and severity of infections.

Iron Absorption:

Vitamin C facilitates the absorption of non-heme iron, the type of iron found in plant-based sources. It converts iron into a more absorbable form, enhancing its uptake in the intestine.

This property of Vitamin C is particularly important for individuals following a vegetarian or vegan diet, as plant-based sources of iron may not be as readily absorbed without the presence of Vitamin C.

Antiviral Activity:

Vitamin C has demonstrated antiviral properties, potentially aiding in the prevention and management of viral infections. It has been studied for its potential benefits in reducing the severity and duration of respiratory tract infections, including the common cold and flu. While Vitamin C cannot cure viral infections, it may support the immune system's response to combat them.

Wound Healing:

Vitamin C plays a crucial role in the wound healing process. It contributes to the synthesis of collagen, the formation of new blood vessels, and the repair of damaged tissues. Adequate Vitamin C levels are essential for proper wound healing, ensuring efficient tissue regeneration and reducing the risk of complications.

Skin Health:

Vitamin C's antioxidant properties and its role in collagen synthesis make it beneficial for skin health. It helps protect the skin against oxidative stress, which can contribute to premature aging and skin damage. Vitamin C also supports the production of collagen, promoting skin elasticity, reducing the appearance of wrinkles, and enhancing overall skin health.

Eye Health:

Vitamin C's antioxidant properties may benefit eye health by protecting against oxidative stress and reducing the risk of age-related macular degeneration (AMD) and cataracts, two common eye conditions that can lead to vision impairment or loss.

Stress Management:

Vitamin C is known to play a role in the body's stress response. During times of stress, Vitamin C levels may become depleted. Adequate intake of Vitamin C helps support the adrenal glands, which produce stress hormones, and helps maintain optimal levels during stressful periods.

General Well-being:

Vitamin C's multifaceted roles and benefits contribute to overall well-being. From its antioxidant protection and collagen synthesis to immune support and various other functions, Vitamin C helps maintain optimal health, vitality, and resilience against various stressors.

Food Sources Rich in Vitamin C

Vitamin C is a vital nutrient that the body cannot produce on its own, making it essential to obtain from dietary sources. Fortunately, a wide array of fruits and vegetables are rich in Vitamin C, allowing us to harness nature's abundance for optimal intake. Let's explore some of the top food sources known for their Vitamin C content:

Citrus Fruits:

They not only provide a refreshing burst of flavor but also offer a significant dose of this essential nutrient.

Consuming these fruits whole or as freshly squeezed juices can contribute to meeting your daily Vitamin C needs.

Berries:

Berries, including strawberries, blueberries, raspberries, and blackberries, are packed with antioxidants and Vitamin C. These colorful gems make a delicious addition to various dishes, including smoothies, yogurt bowls, salads, and desserts, while providing a boost of Vitamin C and other health-promoting compounds.

Kiwi:

Its vibrant green flesh is loaded with nutrients and antioxidants, including Vitamin C, making it a nutritious and delicious addition to your diet. Enjoy it on its own, slice it into fruit salads, or blend it into smoothies for a refreshing treat.

Bell Peppers:

Bell peppers, especially the red and yellow varieties, are not only crunchy and flavorful but also rich in Vitamin C. These versatile vegetables can be enjoyed raw in salads, sliced and dipped in hummus, or cooked in stir-fries and other dishes to enhance their Vitamin C content.

Guava:

Just one guava fruit can provide more than double the recommended daily intake of Vitamin C. This tropical delight can be eaten as is or used in smoothies, jams, and other culinary creations.

Papaya:

Papaya is not only a delicious tropical fruit but also a great source of Vitamin C. Its sweet and juicy flesh is not only refreshing but also provides a substantial amount of this essential nutrient. Enjoy papaya as a standalone fruit, add it to fruit salads, or blend it into smoothies for a tropical twist.

Pineapple:

Pineapple is a tropical fruit known for its unique taste and juiciness. Whether enjoyed fresh, grilled, or incorporated into fruit salads and salsas, pineapple can add a tangy sweetness along with a dose of Vitamin C to your meals.

Leafy Greens:

Leafy greens, such as spinach, kale, and Swiss chard, may not be the first foods that come to mind when you think of Vitamin C, but they still offer a notable amount. These nutrient-packed greens can be enjoyed in salads, sautéed as a side dish, or added to smoothies to boost your Vitamin C intake.

Broccoli:

Broccoli is a cruciferous vegetable that is not only rich in fiber and other essential nutrients but also a good source of Vitamin C. Enjoy it steamed, roasted, or added to stir-fries and salads to reap its health benefits, including its Vitamin C content.

Tomatoes:

They are versatile and can be used in salads, sauces, sandwiches, and various other dishes, making them a convenient way to incorporate Vitamin C into your meals.

Recommended Daily Intake of Vitamin C

Determining the appropriate daily intake of Vitamin C is crucial for maintaining optimal health and reaping the benefits of this essential nutrient. The recommended intake can vary depending on age, sex, life stage, and overall health. Let's explore the general guidelines for daily Vitamin C intake:

Adults:

For most adults, the recommended daily intake of Vitamin C ranges from 75 to 90 milligrams (mg) for women and 90 mg for men. However, certain factors may warrant higher intakes. For example, smokers are advised to consume an additional 35 mg of Vitamin C per day due to increased oxidative stress from smoking.

Pregnancy and Breastfeeding:

During pregnancy and lactation, the body's requirements for Vitamin C increase to support maternal and fetal health. Pregnant women are recommended to consume 85 mg of Vitamin C per day, while breastfeeding women are advised to increase their intake to 120 mg per day.

Infants and Children:

The recommended daily intake of Vitamin C for infants and children varies based on age:

Infants (up to 6 months): 40 mg/day

Infants (7-12 months): 50 mg/day

Children (1-3 years): 15 mg/day

Children (4-8 years): 25 mg/day

Children (9-13 years): 45 mg/day

Adolescents (14-18 years): 65-75 mg/day

Individual Needs and Health Conditions:

It's important to note that individual needs may vary based on specific health conditions or circumstances. In some cases, individuals may require higher intakes of Vitamin C. For example, individuals with certain chronic diseases, smokers, people under high physical or psychological stress, and those recovering from surgery or illness may benefit from increased Vitamin C intake.

Food Sources and Supplementation:

Meeting the recommended daily intake of Vitamin C can be achieved through a well-balanced diet rich in Vitamin C-containing foods. As mentioned earlier, fruits and vegetables such as citrus fruits, berries, kiwi, bell peppers, and leafy greens are excellent sources of Vitamin C. However, in some cases, supplementation may be necessary, especially for individuals who have difficulty meeting their Vitamin C needs through diet alone. Supplements are available in various forms, including tablets, capsules, and powders, and should be used under professional guidance.

Signs of Vitamin C Deficiency

Vitamin C deficiency, also known as scurvy, can have significant implications for overall health. Recognizing the signs and symptoms of Vitamin C deficiency is crucial for timely intervention and ensuring adequate intake of this essential nutrient. Here are some common signs that may indicate a deficiency:

Fatigue and Weakness:

Feeling constantly tired and experiencing unexplained weakness or fatigue can be early signs of Vitamin C deficiency. Vitamin C plays a vital role in energy production and the absorption of iron, which is necessary for the transport of oxygen to body tissues. Inadequate Vitamin C levels can impair these processes, leading to reduced energy levels and overall feelings of weakness.

Easy Bruising and Slow Wound Healing:

Vitamin C is essential for the production of collagen, a protein involved in wound healing and maintaining the integrity of blood vessels. A deficiency in Vitamin C can lead to weakened blood vessels, resulting in easy bruising and slower healing of wounds. Delayed healing of cuts, bruises, or injuries may be indicative of insufficient Vitamin C levels.

Dry and Damaged Skin:

Vitamin C is involved in the synthesis of collagen, which is crucial for maintaining healthy skin. A deficiency in Vitamin C can result in dry, rough, or scaly skin. Additionally, individuals with low Vitamin C levels may experience an increased susceptibility to skin damage, such as skin bruising or the development of small, pinpoint-sized red or purple spots on the skin known as petechiae.

Joint and Muscle Pain:

Inadequate Vitamin C levels can affect the health of connective tissues, including those found in joints and muscles. Joint pain, muscle aches, and stiffness may be indicative of Vitamin C deficiency. These symptoms can significantly impact mobility and overall quality of life.

Weakened Immune System:

A deficiency in this essential nutrient can compromise the immune system, making individuals more susceptible to infections, frequent colds, and other respiratory illnesses.

Poor Oral Health:

Vitamin C deficiency can have negative effects on oral health. It can contribute to gum disease, tooth loss, and impaired dental health. Individuals with low Vitamin C levels may experience loose teeth, gum infections, and delayed wound healing after dental procedures.

Mood Changes and Depression:

Emerging research suggests a potential link between Vitamin C deficiency and mood disorders, including depression. Low Vitamin C levels may contribute to altered neurotransmitter function and imbalances in brain chemistry, affecting mental well-being and mood stability.

3.6 Vitamin C Supplements

While a balanced diet rich in Vitamin C-containing foods is the ideal way to meet your daily needs, certain situations may warrant the use of Vitamin C supplements. Let's explore the key aspects of Vitamin C supplementation:

Supplement Formulations:

Vitamin C supplements are available in various forms, including tablets, capsules, powders, chewable, and liquid formulations. These different forms offer convenience and flexibility in choosing a supplement that suits your preferences and needs.

Dosage Considerations:

The appropriate dosage of Vitamin C supplements depends on individual factors such as age, sex, health status, and specific needs. The recommended dietary allowance (RDA) for Vitamin C varies from 75 to 90 mg for adults, but higher intakes may be warranted in certain circumstances. Consulting with healthcare professionals or registered dietitians can provide personalized guidance on the optimal dosage for your individual needs.

Absorption and Bioavailability:

Vitamin C supplements are generally well-absorbed by the body. However, absorption rates may vary depending on the supplement form, dosage, and individual factors. Higher doses of Vitamin C are often excreted in the urine, which limits the extent of absorption.

Timing of Supplement Intake:

Vitamin C supplements can be taken at any time of the day, with or without food. However, if you experience gastrointestinal discomfort, taking the supplement with a meal may help reduce potential digestive issues. Spread out the dosage throughout the day to maintain a steady supply of Vitamin C in your system.

Interactions and Precautions:

Vitamin C supplements are generally safe for most individuals when consumed within the recommended dosage limits. However, certain individuals or medical conditions may require caution. For example, individuals with a history of kidney stones or certain medical conditions should consult healthcare professionals before taking high-dose Vitamin C supplements. Additionally, Vitamin C supplements may interact with certain medications, such as blood-thinning medications or chemotherapy drugs. It's important to disclose all medications and medical conditions to healthcare professionals before starting any new supplement regimen.

Chapter four

Iodine

Iodine is an essential trace mineral that plays a critical role in maintaining optimal health and well-being. It is an integral component of thyroid hormones, which regulate metabolism, growth, development, and various physiological processes in the body. In this article, we will explore the importance of iodine, its sources, functions, recommended intake, and potential health implications of deficiency or excess.

Functions of Iodine:

Iodine is primarily known for its role in thyroid function. It is necessary for the synthesis of thyroid hormones, including thyroxin (T4) and triiodothyronine (T3), which are essential for regulating metabolism, body temperature, heart rate, growth, and development. These hormones are particularly critical during pregnancy, infancy, and childhood for proper brain development and growth.

Sources of Iodine:

Iodine is found naturally in certain foods and is also present in iodized salt. Seafood, including fish and seaweed, is a rich source of iodine. Other sources include dairy products, eggs, and some fruits and vegetables, although the iodine content may vary depending on the soil in which they are grown. In regions where soil iodine levels are low, iodized salt or iodine supplements may be necessary to ensure adequate intake.

Recommended Daily Intake:

The recommended daily intake of iodine varies across different age groups and life stages. The following are general guidelines:

Infants (0-6 months): 110-130 micrograms (mcg)

Infants (7-12 months): 130 mcg

Children (1-8 years): 90-120 mcg

Children (9-13 years): 120 mcg

Adolescents (14-18 years): 150 mcg

Adults (19 years and older): 150 mcg

Pregnancy: 220 mcg

Lactation: 290 mcg

Iodine Deficiency:

Inadequate iodine intake can lead to iodine deficiency, which is a significant global health concern, particularly in regions where soil and food iodine levels are low. Iodine deficiency can have severe consequences, including impaired thyroid function, goiter (enlargement of the thyroid gland), and developmental issues, particularly in infants and children. Pregnant women with iodine deficiency are at a higher risk of complications, including miscarriage, stillbirth, and intellectual impairments in their children.

Health Risks of Excess Iodine:

While iodine deficiency is a concern, excessive iodine intake can also have adverse effects. Consuming very high levels of iodine, typically through supplements or certain foods, may disrupt thyroid function and lead to hyperthyroidism or hypothyroidism. It is important to stay within the recommended intake range and avoid self-supplementation without healthcare professional guidance.

Iodine and Thyroid Health:

Iodine is crucial for proper thyroid function. Both iodine deficiency and excess can disrupt thyroid hormone production, leading to thyroid disorders. In regions with severe iodine deficiency, endemic goiter may develop, characterized by the enlargement of the thyroid gland in an attempt to compensate for inadequate iodine intake. On the other hand, excess iodine intake can contribute to the development of autoimmune thyroid diseases, such as Hashimoto's thyroiditis or Grave's disease.

Functions and Importance of Iodine

Iodine, an essential trace mineral, is fundamental to maintaining optimal health and functioning of the human body. Let's delve into the functions and importance of iodine in detail:

Thyroid Hormone Synthesis:

Iodine is a vital component of thyroid hormones, including thyroxin (T4) and triiodothyronine (T3). These hormones are synthesized in the thyroid gland and play a central role in regulating metabolism, growth, and development. Iodine is incorporated into the structure of these hormones, ensuring their proper formation and function.

Metabolic Regulation:

The thyroid hormones, influenced by iodine, play a key role in regulating the body's metabolic rate. They help determine the speed at which cells convert nutrients into energy, affecting various bodily functions, including digestion, heart rate, body temperature, and weight management. Adequate iodine levels are essential for maintaining a healthy metabolic balance.

Growth and Development:

Iodine is crucial for normal growth and development, especially during fetal and early childhood stages. Adequate iodine intake is essential for proper brain development, cognitive function, and overall physical growth.

Reproductive Health:

Iodine plays a role in reproductive health for both men and women. In women, iodine is important for maintaining regular menstrual cycles and optimal fertility. During pregnancy, iodine is critical for the healthy development of the fetus, including proper brain development. Adequate iodine levels are necessary for supporting a healthy pregnancy and preventing complications such as miscarriage, stillbirth, or impaired cognitive function in the child.

Cognitive Function:

Iodine is essential for optimal cognitive function, including memory, attention, and overall mental performance. Adequate iodine intake during early development and throughout life is associated with better cognitive abilities, particularly in children. Iodine deficiency can impair cognitive function, leading to learning difficulties and lower IQ levels.

Regulation of Metabolism:

Iodine is involved in the synthesis of various enzymes that are essential for the metabolism of carbohydrates, fats, and proteins. It aids in the breakdown and utilization of these macronutrients for energy production and ensures their proper utilization within cells.

Thyroid Gland Health:

Adequate iodine levels are essential for maintaining the health and proper functioning of the thyroid gland itself. Iodine deficiency can lead to the enlargement of the thyroid gland, known as goiter, as the gland attempts to compensate for the lack of iodine. Ensuring sufficient iodine intake helps prevent thyroid disorders and promotes the overall well-being of the gland.

Antioxidant Properties:

Iodine exhibits antioxidant properties, protecting cells from damage caused by free radicals. It helps neutralize these harmful molecules, reducing oxidative stress and preventing cellular damage. This antioxidant effect of iodine contributes to overall health and may help prevent chronic diseases associated with oxidative stress.

Immune System Support:

Iodine plays a role in supporting a healthy immune system. It helps regulate the activity of immune cells and enhances the body's defense mechanisms against infections and diseases. Adequate iodine levels are important for optimal immune function and overall immune response.

Food Sources:

Iodine can be obtained from various dietary sources. Seafood, including fish, shellfish, and seaweed, is particularly rich in iodine. Dairy products, eggs, and iodized salt are also sources of iodine. However, the iodine content in plant-based foods depends on the iodine content of the soil in which they are grown.

Ensuring Adequate Iodine Intake:

Maintaining adequate iodine levels is crucial for overall health and well-being. In areas where iodine deficiency is prevalent, iodized salt is an effective method of increasing iodine intake. However, it's important to note that excessive iodine intake can also have adverse effects, so it's crucial to strike a balance.

Dietary Sources of Iodine

Iodine is an essential trace mineral that the body requires for various functions, including thyroid hormone synthesis, growth, and cognitive development. While the human body cannot produce iodine on its own, it can be obtained through dietary sources. Let's explore some of the key dietary sources of iodine:

Seafood:

Seafood, particularly seaweed and saltwater fish, is one of the richest sources of iodine. Seaweed, such as kelp, nori, and wakame, contains exceptionally high iodine levels due to its ability to absorb iodine from seawater. Fish like cod, tuna, shrimp, and haddock also contain significant amounts of iodine. Including seafood in your diet can provide a natural and reliable source of iodine.

Dairy Products:

Dairy products, including milk, yogurt, and cheese, are good sources of iodine. This is mainly due to the iodine content in the cattle feed and the use of iodine-based sanitizers during milk processing. However, the iodine content can vary depending on the region and farming practices.

Eggs:

Eggs are a moderate source of iodine, with the iodine content varying depending on the diet of the hens. Eggs from hens fed with iodine-rich feed or iodine-fortified feed can provide a good source of dietary iodine. Including eggs in your diet can contribute to overall iodine intake.

Iodized Salt:

Iodized salt, which is regular table salt fortified with iodine, is a widely available and convenient source of iodine. It is a common strategy used to prevent iodine deficiency in regions where iodine deficiency is prevalent. Using iodized salt in cooking or as a seasoning can help meet your daily iodine needs. However, it's important to note that excessive salt consumption should be avoided due to its potential impact on blood pressure.

Seaweed and Seaweed Products:

Seaweed, such as kelp, nori, and dulse, is not only a rich source of iodine but also provides various other nutrients and minerals.

Iodine-Fortified Foods:

In some regions, certain foods are fortified with iodine to address iodine deficiency. This includes iodine-fortified bread, cereals, and other processed foods. Checking food labels for "iodized" or "fortified with iodine" can help identify products that contribute to iodine intake.

Achieving Adequate Iodine Intake:

Maintaining adequate iodine intake is crucial for overall health and well-being. The recommended daily intake of iodine varies based on age, sex, and life stage. In regions where iodine deficiency is prevalent, consuming iodized salt and including iodine-rich foods in the diet can help ensure sufficient iodine intake. However, it's essential to strike a balance and avoid excessive iodine intake, which can have adverse effects.

Consulting healthcare professionals or registered dietitians can provide personalized guidance on iodine intake based on individual needs, geographical location, and specific health conditions. Regular monitoring of iodine levels through urine or blood tests can help ensure appropriate iodine intake and prevent deficiencies or excesses.

Recommended Daily Intake of Iodine

Determining the appropriate daily intake of iodine is crucial for maintaining optimal health and ensuring the proper functioning of the thyroid gland. The recommended intake can vary depending on age, sex, life stage, and specific health conditions. Let's explore the general guidelines for daily iodine intake:

Adults:

For most adults, the recommended daily intake of iodine ranges from 150 to 290 micrograms (mcg). However, pregnant and breastfeeding women have higher iodine requirements. Pregnant women are advised to consume 220 mcg of iodine per day, while breastfeeding women are recommended to increase their intake to 290 mcg per day.

Infants and Children:

The recommended daily intake of iodine for infants and children varies based on age:

Infants (up to 6 months): 110 mcg/day

Infants (7-12 months): 130 mcg/day

Children (1-8 years): 90 mcg/day

Children (9-13 years): 120 mcg/day

Adolescents (14-18 years): 150 mcg/day

Pregnancy and Breastfeeding:

During pregnancy and lactation, iodine requirements increase significantly to support maternal and fetal health. Adequate iodine intake is crucial for proper brain development and growth of the baby. Pregnant women should consult healthcare professionals to ensure they meet their specific iodine needs, as it may require additional supplementation.

Individual Needs and Health Conditions:

It's important to note that individual iodine needs may vary based on specific health conditions or circumstances. Some individuals may require higher intakes of iodine. For example, individuals with thyroid disorders or those living in regions with iodine-deficient soils may require iodine supplementation or higher iodine intake. Consulting healthcare professionals can provide personalized guidance on the optimal iodine intake for individual needs and health status.

Iodine from Food and Supplements:

Iodine can be obtained from various dietary sources, including seafood, dairy products, eggs, and iodized salt. In regions where iodine deficiency is prevalent, using iodized salt in cooking or seasoning can be an effective way to increase iodine intake. In some cases, iodine supplements may be necessary to ensure adequate intake, especially for individuals who have difficulty meeting their iodine needs through diet alone. However, supplementation should be done under healthcare professional guidance to avoid excessive iodine intake.

Ensuring Adequate Iodine Intake:

Maintaining adequate iodine levels is crucial for overall health, particularly for proper thyroid function and cognitive development. However, it's important to strike a balance, as excessive iodine intake can also have adverse effects. Monitoring iodine levels through urine or blood tests can help ensure appropriate iodine intake and prevent deficiencies or excesses.

In regions where iodine deficiency is prevalent, public health initiatives may include iodized salt programs to address the issue. Checking food labels for iodine content, incorporating iodine-rich foods into the diet, and following healthcare professional recommendations can help achieve optimal iodine intake.

Iodine Deficiency Disorders

As a trace mineral, iodine plays a critical role in the functioning of the human body. Both from a chemical and medical perspective, understanding iodine deficiency disorders (IDD) sheds light on the profound impact of iodine insufficiency.

Let's delve into this topic, embracing both the language of chemistry and medicine:

Chemical Perspective:

From a chemical perspective, iodine deficiency disrupts the homeostasis of thyroid hormones, which are critical for regulating various physiological processes. Thyroxine (T4) and triiodothyronine (T3) play essential roles in cellular metabolism, growth, development, and energy balance. These hormones contain iodine atoms bound to the amino acid tyrosine within the thyroglobulin molecule, forming the building blocks of thyroid hormones. Insufficient iodine availability hampers the synthesis of T4 and T3, compromising their production and leading to imbalances in thyroid hormone levels.

From a chemical standpoint, iodine deficiency arises when the body lacks an adequate supply of this essential element. Iodine is an essential component of thyroid hormones, including thyroxin (T4) and triiodothyronine (T3). These hormones contain three and four iodine atoms, respectively, which confer their biochemical activity. The availability of iodine is critical for proper hormone synthesis, as the thyroid gland selectively incorporates iodine into thyroglobulin, a precursor protein that undergoes enzymatic conversion to produce active thyroid hormones. Insufficient iodine limits the production of these hormones, leading to imbalances and disruptions in various bodily functions.

Medical Perspective:

In the medical realm, iodine deficiency disorders encompass a range of conditions resulting from inadequate iodine intake. The most well-known disorder is goiter, characterized by the enlargement of the thyroid gland. In response to insufficient iodine, the thyroid gland enlarges in an attempt to compensate for the reduced iodine availability. This compensatory response, driven by the release of thyroid-stimulating hormone (TSH) from the pituitary gland, leads to the visible swelling of the neck area.

Medical Perspective:

Iodine deficiency disorders have varying clinical presentations and severity, depending on the duration and severity of the deficiency.

Besides goiter and cretinism, there are other manifestations of iodine deficiency:

Hypothyroidism:

Prolonged iodine deficiency can result in an underactive thyroid gland, leading to hypothyroidism. Symptoms may include fatigue, weight gain, and sensitivity to cold, dry skin, hair loss, and constipation. Hypothyroidism can negatively impact overall health and well-being if left untreated.

Intellectual and Developmental Impairments:

Inadequate iodine during fetal and early childhood development can have profound effects on cognitive function and physical growth. Children born to iodine-deficient mothers are at a higher risk of intellectual impairments, lower IQ, learning difficulties, and stunted growth. The severity of these impairments depends on the extent and duration of iodine deficiency.

Increased Risk of Pregnancy Complications:

Iodine deficiency in pregnant women can lead to various complications, including miscarriage, stillbirth, preterm birth, and increased maternal and infant mortality rates. It can also result in maternal and neonatal thyroid dysfunction, which can have long-term consequences on both the mother and the baby.

Impaired Immune Function:

Adequate iodine levels are crucial for optimal immune function. Iodine deficiency compromises the immune system, making individuals more susceptible to infections and impairing the body's ability to fight off pathogens effectively.

Addressing Iodine Deficiency:

Addressing iodine deficiency requires a multi-faceted approach involving public health initiatives, dietary interventions, and education:

Universal Salt Iodization (USI):

Implementing USI programs, where iodized salt is made widely available and affordable, has proven to be a successful strategy in addressing iodine deficiency on a population level. This approach ensures that individuals receive adequate iodine through regular consumption of iodized salt.

Food Fortification:

Fortifying staple foods, such as flour, with iodine is another effective method to increase iodine intake, especially in regions where salt consumption is limited. This approach reaches a broader population, including those who do not regularly consume iodized salt.

Health Education:

Raising awareness about the importance of iodine and its food sources can help individuals make informed choices to ensure adequate intake. Education campaigns targeting pregnant women, healthcare providers, and the general public can play a crucial role in preventing and managing iodine deficiency disorders.

Iodine Supplementation:

In areas where iodine deficiency remains prevalent, iodine supplementation, in the form of tablets or drops, may be necessary for vulnerable populations, such as pregnant women and young children. Supplementation should be done under healthcare professional guidance to ensure appropriate dosage and minimize the risk of excessive iodine intake.

A Multidisciplinary Approach:

The understanding and management of iodine deficiency disorders require a multidisciplinary approach, drawing on the fields of chemistry and medicine. Combining chemical knowledge of iodine's role in hormone synthesis with medical expertise in diagnosing and treating related disorders empowers us to address this global health concern effectively.

Iodine Supplementation

Iodine supplementation is a targeted approach to address iodine deficiency, ensuring individuals receive adequate levels of this essential trace mineral. This intervention plays a crucial role in preventing and correcting iodine deficiencies, particularly in areas where dietary iodine intake is insufficient. Let's explore iodine supplementation in detail:

Purpose of Iodine Supplementation:

Iodine supplementation aims to provide individuals with an additional source of iodine to meet their daily requirements. It is commonly used in regions where iodine deficiency is prevalent or for specific populations at higher risk of deficiency, such as pregnant women and young children. Supplementation can help prevent the development of iodine deficiency disorders and support overall health and well-being.

Types of Iodine Supplements:

Iodine supplements are available in different forms, including tablets, capsules, drops, and liquid solutions. The most common forms include:

a. Potassium Iodide (KI): This is the most commonly used form of iodine supplementation. Potassium iodide is a stable compound that provides a concentrated source of iodine.

b. Iodine Complexes: These supplements combine iodine with other compounds, such as amino acids or minerals, to enhance absorption or stability. Examples include iodine combined with tyrosine or iodine complexes with minerals like selenium or zinc.

Recommended Dosage:

The recommended dosage of iodine supplements varies depending on the age, sex, life stage, and specific health conditions. Here are some general guidelines:

a. Adults: The recommended daily dosage for most adults is typically around 150 to 290 micrograms (mcg) of iodine. However, pregnant and breastfeeding women have higher iodine requirements, with recommended dosages ranging from 220 to 290 mcg per day.

b. Infants and Children: The recommended dosage for infants and children varies based on age. It ranges from 110 mcg/day for infants up to 6 months, to 150 mcg/day for adolescents aged 14 to 18 years.

c. Specific Conditions: Individuals with certain health conditions, such as thyroid disorders or those residing in iodine-deficient areas, may require higher iodine supplementation dosages. Healthcare professionals can provide personalized recommendations based on individual needs and circumstances.

Health Professional Guidance:

It is important to consult with healthcare professionals, such as doctors or registered dietitians, before starting iodine supplementation. They can assess individual iodine status, evaluate specific health conditions, and provide tailored recommendations on dosage and duration of supplementation.

Timing of Supplementation:

The timing of iodine supplementation can vary. It is generally recommended to take iodine supplements with meals to enhance absorption and minimize potential gastrointestinal side effects. However, the specific timing may depend on the supplement formulation and individual preferences.

Monitoring Iodine Levels:

Regular monitoring of iodine levels is crucial for individuals on iodine supplementation. This can be done through urine or blood tests to ensure that iodine intake remains within the appropriate range. Monitoring helps healthcare professionals adjust supplementation dosages as needed to prevent both deficiency and excessive iodine intake.

Potential Side Effects and Precautions:

While iodine supplementation is generally safe when taken within recommended dosages, excessive iodine intake can have adverse effects. It is important to follow healthcare professional recommendations and avoid self-supplementation without appropriate guidance. Individuals with certain health conditions, such as autoimmune thyroid disease or iodine sensitivity, should exercise caution and consult healthcare professionals before starting supplementation.

Chapter five

Synergistic Effects of Vitamin D, Vitamin C, and Iodine

The combination of vitamin D, vitamin C, and iodine creates a potent nutrient triad that offers synergistic effects and significant health benefits. Individually, these nutrients play crucial roles in various physiological processes, but when combined, their interactions can enhance their individual functions and deliver remarkable health outcomes.

Let's explore the synergistic effects of vitamin D, vitamin C, and iodine and how they work together to support overall health and well-being:

Immune System Boost:

Vitamin D, vitamin C, and iodine all contribute to a robust immune system, and their synergistic effects can have a profound impact on immune function. Vitamin D plays a crucial role in immune cell regulation and the production of antimicrobial peptides, while vitamin C acts as a potent antioxidant, protecting immune cells from oxidative stress.

Iodine supports immune cell activity and enhances the body's defense mechanisms against infections. Together, these nutrients support a healthy immune response and help protect against pathogens, reducing the risk of infections and promoting overall wellness.

Bone Health and Calcium Absorption:

Vitamin D and iodine work synergistically to promote bone health and calcium absorption. Vitamin D aids in the absorption of calcium from the diet and helps maintain adequate levels of calcium in the bloodstream. Iodine is essential for the production of thyroid hormones, which play a role in bone metabolism. Together, these nutrients support proper bone mineralization, density, and strength, reducing the risk of osteoporosis and promoting skeletal health.

Cognitive Function and Brain Health:

Vitamin D, vitamin C, and iodine all contribute to optimal cognitive function and brain health. Vitamin D receptors are present in various areas of the brain, and vitamin D deficiency has been associated with cognitive impairment and an increased risk of neurodegenerative diseases.

Vitamin C acts as an antioxidant and supports the synthesis of neurotransmitters, which are essential for brain function. Iodine is crucial for proper brain development, particularly during fetal and early childhood stages. By working synergistically, these nutrients support cognitive performance, memory, and overall brain health.

Antioxidant Defense and Cellular Protection:

Vitamin C and iodine are powerful antioxidants, while vitamin D also exhibits antioxidant properties. Antioxidants play a crucial role in neutralizing harmful free radicals and reducing oxidative stress, which can damage cells and contribute to aging and chronic diseases. The synergistic effects of these nutrients enhance the body's antioxidant defense system, protecting cells from oxidative damage and supporting overall cellular health.

Thyroid Function and Hormonal Balance:

Iodine is essential for the production of thyroid hormones, which regulate metabolism and play a crucial role in maintaining hormonal balance. Vitamin D is involved in the regulation of thyroid function and can modulate the expression of thyroid-related genes.

Vitamin C supports the synthesis and conversion of thyroid hormones. Together, these nutrients support optimal thyroid function, ensuring proper metabolism, hormone production, and overall endocrine health.

Skin Health and Protection:

Vitamin D, vitamin C, and iodine contribute to healthy skin and protect against various skin conditions. Vitamin D has been linked to skin health, and its deficiency has been associated with skin problems such as psoriasis and eczema.

Iodine's antimicrobial properties help prevent bacterial overgrowth on the skin, supporting overall skin health. By working synergistically, these nutrients promote healthy, vibrant skin and protect against skin damage and aging.

Mood Regulation and Mental Well-being:

Vitamin D, vitamin C, and iodine all play a role in mood regulation and mental well-being. Vitamin D receptors are found in areas of the brain associated with mood and emotional regulation, and vitamin D deficiency has been linked to an increased risk of depression and other mood disorders. Vitamin C is involved in the synthesis of neurotransmitters that influence mood and mental health.

Cardiovascular Health:

Vitamin D, vitamin C, and iodine collectively contribute to cardiovascular health. Vitamin D deficiency has been associated with an increased risk of cardiovascular diseases, including hypertension and heart disease. Vitamin C acts as an antioxidant and supports healthy blood vessel function. Iodine helps regulate heart rate and blood pressure. Together, these nutrients support a healthy cardiovascular system, promoting optimal heart function and reducing the risk of cardiovascular diseases.

Energy Production and Vitality:

Vitamin D, vitamin C, and iodine all play a role in energy production and overall vitality. Vitamin D influences mitochondrial function, the powerhouse of the cell responsible for energy production. Vitamin C is involved in the synthesis of carnitine, a molecule necessary for the transport of fatty acids into the mitochondria for energy production. Iodine supports metabolism and the efficient conversion of food into energy. By working synergistically, these nutrients contribute to optimal energy levels, reducing fatigue, and promoting overall vitality.

Incorporating the synergistic effects of vitamin D, vitamin C, and iodine into daily nutrition can have profound implications for overall health and well-being. While a balanced diet that includes nutrient-rich foods is crucial, supplementation may be necessary to ensure adequate levels of these essential nutrients. As always, it is important to consult with healthcare professionals or registered dietitians for personalized recommendations and guidance on appropriate dosages and combinations of supplements.

Immune System Support

A robust immune system is essential for defending the body against pathogens and maintaining optimal health. Vitamin D, vitamin C, and iodine play integral roles in supporting immune function, and their collective power can provide significant support to the immune system.

Let's explore how these nutrients contribute to immune system support and the synergistic effects they offer:

Vitamin D and Immune Function:

Vitamin D is crucial for immune system regulation and defense against pathogens. It supports the production of antimicrobial peptides, such as cathelicidin and defensins, which have antimicrobial properties and help destroy invading microorganisms. Vitamin D also modulates the activity of immune cells, such as T cells, B cells, and macrophages, enhancing their response to infections. Adequate vitamin D levels are associated with reduced susceptibility to respiratory tract infections, autoimmune diseases, and other immune-related disorders.

Vitamin C and Immune Enhancement:

Vitamin C is well-known for its immune-enhancing properties. It acts as a powerful antioxidant, protecting immune cells from oxidative stress and supporting their optimal function. Vitamin C stimulates the production of white blood cells, including lymphocytes and phagocytes, which are essential for immune defense.

It also enhances the activity of natural killer cells, which target and destroy infected cells. Additionally, vitamin C supports the production of antibodies, strengthening the immune response. Adequate vitamin C levels are associated with reduced severity and duration of common cold symptoms and enhanced immune function.

Iodine and Immune Modulation:

Iodine contributes to immune system modulation and defense against infections. It supports the activity of various immune cells, including natural killer cells, macrophages, and neutrophils, which are crucial for combating pathogens. Iodine's antimicrobial properties help inhibit the growth of bacteria, viruses, and fungi, reducing the risk of infections. Additionally, iodine supports the production of cytokines, which are signaling molecules involved in immune system coordination and regulation.

Synergistic Effects:

When vitamin D, vitamin C, and iodine work together, they offer synergistic effects that can further enhance immune system support. Vitamin D enhances the absorption and utilization of vitamin C, allowing for its optimal antioxidant activity and immune-enhancing effects. Vitamin C, in turn, supports vitamin D metabolism and activation, ensuring adequate vitamin D levels for immune system regulation. Iodine's immune-modulating properties complement the effects of vitamin D and vitamin C, further strengthening the immune response.

Antioxidant Defense:

Vitamin C and iodine both possess antioxidant properties, which are crucial for immune system support. Antioxidants neutralize harmful free radicals, preventing oxidative stress and cellular damage. By protecting immune cells from oxidative damage, vitamin C and iodine help maintain their optimal function and viability. This antioxidant defense also contributes to reducing inflammation, supporting immune system balance and effectiveness.

Respiratory Health:

The collective action of vitamin D, vitamin C, and iodine supports respiratory health, making them particularly relevant in defending against respiratory infections. Vitamin D helps regulate the immune response in the respiratory tract, reducing the risk of respiratory infections and the severity of symptoms. Vitamin C enhances immune function in the respiratory system, reducing inflammation and protecting against oxidative damage. Iodine's antimicrobial properties help combat pathogens in the respiratory tract, supporting healthy lung function and reducing the risk of respiratory infections.

Stress Response and Immunity:

Vitamin C and iodine are involved in the body's stress response and immune function regulation. During times of stress, the body's demand for vitamin C and iodine increases. Adequate levels of these nutrients are necessary for optimal immune system function and adaptation to stress. Supplementing with vitamin C and iodine during periods of increased stress can support immune resilience and overall well-being.

Overall Health and Wellness:

By supporting immune function, vitamin D, vitamin C, and iodine contribute to maintaining optimal health, reducing the risk of infections, and promoting vitality. These nutrients also offer additional benefits beyond immune support, including cardiovascular health, cognitive function, antioxidant defense, and bone health.

Chapter Six

Testing and Monitoring Nutrient Levels

Testing and monitoring nutrient levels is a critical aspect of maintaining optimal health and well-being. By assessing the levels of essential nutrients in the body, healthcare professionals can identify deficiencies or imbalances and develop targeted interventions to restore or optimize nutrient status. Let's explore the importance of testing and monitoring nutrient levels and the methodologies involved:

Assessing Nutritional Status:

Testing nutrient levels provides valuable insights into an individual's nutritional status. It helps identify deficiencies, excesses, or imbalances of key nutrients that can impact overall health and various physiological processes. By evaluating nutrient levels, healthcare professionals can determine if dietary adjustments, lifestyle modifications, or targeted supplementation are necessary to achieve optimal nutrient status.

Personalized Nutrition:

Testing nutrient levels enables healthcare professionals to develop personalized nutrition plans tailored to individual needs. By understanding a person's nutrient status, healthcare professionals can recommend specific dietary changes or nutrient supplementation strategies to address deficiencies or optimize nutrient intake. This personalized approach ensures that individuals receive the right nutrients in the right amounts, promoting overall health and preventing nutrient-related health conditions.

Identifying Deficiencies and Imbalances:

Nutrient testing helps identify specific nutrient deficiencies or imbalances that may be contributing to health issues or symptoms. For example, testing vitamin D levels can reveal a deficiency that may be linked to bone health problems or immune system dysfunction. Similarly, testing vitamin B12 levels can diagnose deficiencies associated with anemia or neurological issues. Identifying these deficiencies or imbalances allows healthcare professionals to implement targeted interventions to address the underlying causes.

Monitoring Treatment Effectiveness:

Nutrient testing plays a crucial role in monitoring the effectiveness of interventions aimed at correcting nutrient deficiencies or imbalances. Regular monitoring allows healthcare professionals to track changes in nutrient levels over time and assess the impact of dietary modifications or supplementation. By monitoring nutrient levels, adjustments can be made to treatment plans to ensure optimal nutrient status is achieved and maintained.

Preventing Chronic Diseases:

Nutrient testing can help identify risk factors for chronic diseases related to nutrient deficiencies or imbalances. For example, testing for blood glucose levels can assess the risk of developing diabetes, while testing cholesterol levels can evaluate cardiovascular health. By addressing nutrient deficiencies or imbalances early on, individuals can take proactive steps to reduce the risk of developing chronic diseases and promote long-term health.

Testing Methodologies:

Various methodologies are used to test nutrient levels, including blood tests, urine tests, and tissue analysis. Blood tests are commonly used to assess nutrient status as they provide a snapshot of nutrient levels in the bloodstream. Urine tests can measure nutrient excretion and provide insights into nutrient absorption and utilization. In certain cases, tissue analysis, such as hair mineral analysis, can be utilized to assess long-term nutrient status. The choice of testing methodology depends on the specific nutrient being evaluated and the healthcare professional's clinical judgment.

Professional Guidance:

It is essential to seek professional guidance from healthcare professionals or registered dietitians when considering nutrient testing. They have the expertise to interpret test results accurately, provide appropriate recommendations, and develop personalized interventions based on individual needs.

Blood Tests for Vitamin D, Vitamin C, and Iodine

Blood tests serve as valuable tools for assessing the levels of essential nutrients such as vitamin D, vitamin C, and iodine. These tests provide healthcare professionals with quantitative data to evaluate nutrient status, identify deficiencies or imbalances, and guide targeted interventions. Let's explore the specific blood tests used to assess the levels of these nutrients:

Vitamin D Blood Test:

The most common blood test for assessing vitamin D status is the 25-hydroxyvitamin D (25(OH) D) test. It measures the levels of 25(OH) D in the blood, which is the main circulating form of vitamin D. The results are usually reported as Nano grams per milliliter (ng/mL) or nanomoles per liter (nmol/L). The optimal range for vitamin D levels may vary based on individual circumstances and guidelines, but generally, levels above 30 ng/mL (75 nmol/L) are considered desirable for most individuals.

Vitamin C Blood Test:

Measuring vitamin C levels in the blood can be challenging due to its rapid turnover and utilization in the body. However, the plasma ascorbic acid level is often used as an indicator of vitamin C status.

The optimal range for vitamin C levels may vary based on individual circumstances, but a level above 0.6 mg/dL

(34 µmol/L) is generally considered sufficient to prevent deficiency-related health conditions.

Iodine Blood Test:

The urinary iodine concentration (UIC) test is commonly used to assess iodine status. This test measures the amount of iodine excreted in the urine over a specified period. The results are reported as micrograms per liter (µg/L). Optimal ranges for iodine levels may vary depending on age, sex, and specific health considerations. Generally, UIC levels between 100-200 µg/L are considered sufficient for most individuals, although reference ranges can differ in regions with varying iodine intake levels.

It is important to consult with healthcare professionals or registered dietitians to determine the appropriate blood tests for assessing vitamin D, vitamin C, and iodine levels. They can interpret the test results, provide insights into nutrient status, and guide personalized interventions based on individual needs. Nutrient testing should be part of a comprehensive approach to evaluating overall nutritional status and optimizing health outcomes.

Interpreting Test Results

Interpreting test results for nutrient assessments requires a comprehensive understanding of reference ranges, individual circumstances, and clinical judgment. Healthcare professionals play a crucial role in analyzing and interpreting these results to provide meaningful insights into an individual's nutrient status. Let's delve into the key aspects involved in interpreting test results for vitamin D, vitamin C, and iodine:

Reference Ranges:

Reference ranges provide a benchmark for evaluating nutrient levels and comparing them to established standards. These ranges are typically based on population studies and take into account various factors such as age, sex, and health conditions. It is important to note that reference ranges may differ among laboratories or regions due to variations in testing methods and population characteristics. Healthcare professionals use these reference ranges as a guide, but individual circumstances and clinical judgment are also crucial for accurate interpretation.

Optimal vs. Deficient:

When interpreting nutrient test results, the aim is to assess whether nutrient levels fall within optimal ranges or indicate deficiency. Optimal ranges are typically determined based on maintaining adequate physiological function and minimizing the risk of deficiency-related health issues. Deficiency thresholds may vary depending on the nutrient and the specific health condition being evaluated.

Individual Circumstances:

Interpreting test results involves considering individual circumstances that may influence nutrient status. Factors such as age, sex, overall health, pregnancy or lactation, medication use, and underlying medical conditions can impact nutrient requirements and metabolism. For example, vitamin D requirements may be higher for older adults or individuals with malabsorption issues. Healthcare professionals take these factors into account to provide personalized interpretations and recommendations.

Trends and Patterns:

Assessing nutrient status involves examining trends and patterns over time. Single test results may not always provide a comprehensive picture of nutrient status, as levels can vary due to dietary intake, recent supplementation, or other factors. Monitoring nutrient levels over multiple tests allows healthcare professionals to identify consistent trends and patterns, providing a more accurate assessment of nutrient status and guiding appropriate interventions.

Clinical Correlation:

Interpreting nutrient test results requires clinical correlation with an individual's overall health and symptoms. Nutrient deficiencies or imbalances may present with specific clinical manifestations, and healthcare professionals consider these factors when assessing test results. For example, vitamin C deficiency may manifest as symptoms of scurvy, while vitamin D deficiency may present as musculoskeletal pain or increased susceptibility to infections. Clinical correlation helps guide the interpretation of test results and informs appropriate interventions.

Individualized Interventions:

The interpretation of nutrient test results should guide individualized interventions to address deficiencies or optimize nutrient status. Healthcare professionals use their expertise to recommend appropriate dietary modifications, lifestyle changes, or targeted supplementation based on the specific nutrient deficiencies or imbalances identified. The goal is to tailor interventions to each individual's needs, taking into account their overall health, preferences, and other factors that may impact nutrient status.

Incorporating These Nutrients into Your Diet

I am thrilled to share with you the tremendous benefits of incorporating vitamin D, vitamin C, and iodine into your daily diet. By embracing these essential nutrients, you have the power to elevate your health, vitality, and overall well-being. Let me unveil the reasons why integrating these nutrients into your diet is a game-changer:

Empowering Bone Health and Strength:

Vitamin D, commonly referred to as the "sunshine vitamin," plays a pivotal role in bone health. By ensuring an adequate intake of vitamin D, you provide the necessary support for optimal calcium absorption and utilization, enhancing bone mineralization and strength. Strong and resilient bones are the foundation of an active and vibrant life, enabling you to pursue your passions and enjoy a fulfilling existence.

Fortifying Your Immune System:

Vitamin C, renowned for its immune-boosting prowess, empowers your body's defense mechanisms. By incorporating vitamin C-rich foods into your diet, you bolster your immune system, strengthening its ability to ward off infections and safeguard your well-being.

Unleashing Cognitive Clarity and Vitality:

Iodine, often underestimated, holds the key to cognitive vitality. By embracing iodine-rich sources in your diet, you fuel your brain with the essential nutrient it needs for optimal functioning. Iodine supports cognitive development, mental alertness, and overall brain health, allowing you to navigate life's challenges with clarity, focus, and a sharp mind.

Shielding Against Oxidative Stress and Inflammation:

Vitamin D, vitamin C, and iodine are potent antioxidants, standing as your allies in the battle against oxidative stress and inflammation. These remarkable nutrients neutralize harmful free radicals, preventing cellular damage and reducing the risk of chronic diseases. By incorporating them into your diet, you establish a powerful defense system that safeguards your cells, tissues, and organs, promoting longevity, vitality, and graceful aging.

Enhancing Overall Vitality and Well-being:

Integrating these nutrients into your daily diet sets the stage for a life brimming with vitality and well-being. From supporting energy production and hormone regulation to promoting cardiovascular health and balanced metabolism, vitamin D, vitamin C, and iodine contribute to your overall vitality. By nourishing your body with these essential nutrients, you unlock a reservoir of energy, resilience, and joy, enabling you to thrive in all aspects of life.

Remember, embracing these nutrients is not merely about adopting a diet; it is a transformative step towards a life of optimal health, vitality, and fulfillment.

Here are a few tips to ensure a seamless integration into your lifestyle:

+ Variety is key: Explore a wide range of vitamin D, vitamin C, and iodine-rich foods to make your diet vibrant and exciting. From citrus fruits and leafy greens to fatty fish and iodized salt, indulge in a colorful array of nutrient-dense options that tantalize your taste buds and nourish your body.

- Embrace culinary creativity: Experiment with recipes and culinary techniques that incorporate these nutrients. From refreshing citrus salads to delicious seafood dishes, let your culinary creativity take center stage as you discover new and delectable ways to enjoy these health-enhancing nutrients.

- Seek professional guidance: Consult with healthcare professionals or registered dietitians who can provide personalized guidance tailored to your specific needs and goals. They can help you navigate the world of nutrition, offer expert recommendations, and ensure you optimize your nutrient intake effectively.

Dietary Strategies for Increasing Vitamin D, Vitamin C, and Iodine Intake

By incorporating these nutrient-rich foods into your diet, you nourish your body with essential elements that promote optimal health and vitality.

Let's explore the dietary strategies that will empower you to elevate your nutrient intake:

Amplifying Vitamin D Intake:

To enhance your vitamin D levels, consider the following dietary strategies:

a. Embrace the Sun: Engage in moderate sun exposure, preferably during the early morning or late afternoon when the sun's rays are gentle. Aim for approximately 10-15 minutes of sun exposure on bare skin, such as your arms, legs, or face, several times a week. However, be mindful of sun protection practices to prevent overexposure and sunburn.

b. Savor Fatty Fish: Incorporate fatty fish into your diet, such as salmon, mackerel, and sardines. These delicious sources of vitamin D provide a significant boost to your nutrient intake.

c. Fortified Foods: Look for fortified dairy products, including milk, yogurt, and cheese, as well as plant-based milk alternatives fortified with vitamin D. Fortified orange juice and breakfast cereals can also be excellent additions to your diet.

Elevating Vitamin C Intake:

To harness the power of vitamin C, consider the following dietary strategies:

a. Citrus Fruits: Enjoy a variety of citrus fruits, such as oranges, grapefruits, lemons, and limes. These vibrant fruits are not only refreshing but also rich in vitamin C. Add citrus segments to salads, squeeze fresh lemon or lime juice over dishes, or simply enjoy them as a healthy snack.

b. Colorful Berries: Indulge in a rainbow of berries, including strawberries, blueberries, raspberries, and blackberries. These antioxidant-rich fruits are packed with vitamin C, adding a burst of flavor and nutrients to your diet.

c. Abundant Vegetables: Include a variety of vitamin C-rich vegetables in your meals. Bell peppers (especially red and yellow varieties), broccoli, Brussels sprouts, and leafy greens like kale and spinach are excellent choices. Explore different cooking methods, such as stir-frying or roasting, to retain the nutrient content and enhance the flavors.

Enhancing Iodine Intake:

To unlock the potential of iodine, consider the following dietary strategies:

a. Seafood Delights: Embrace the ocean's bounty by incorporating seafood into your diet. Seaweed and algae are exceptional sources of iodine, making them a valuable addition to your meals. Enjoy sushi rolls with seaweed, explore seaweed salads, or experiment with seaweed-based snacks.

b. Iodized Salt: Use iodized salt as a seasoning in your dishes. This common kitchen staple provides a convenient way to enhance your iodine intake. However, it's important to use salt in moderation and balance it with an overall healthy diet.

c. Dairy Products: Include dairy products such as milk, yogurt, and cheese in your diet. These foods often contain iodine, contributing to your overall intake. Choose high-quality, organic options whenever possible.

Meal Planning Tips

By strategizing your meals and making intentional choices, you can nourish your body with the essential nutrients it needs for optimal health and well-being.

Let's explore the meal planning tips aligned with the content of our discussion:

Overview of Essential Nutrients:

Begin your meal planning journey by understanding the importance of vitamin D, vitamin C, and iodine. Recognize that these nutrients are essential for various physiological functions, and their incorporation into your diet will contribute to your overall health and vitality.

Importance of Vitamin D, Vitamin C, and Iodine:

Acknowledge the significance of these nutrients in your meal planning efforts. Understand their roles in bone health, immune support, cognitive function, and cellular protection. By keeping their importance in mind, you can prioritize their inclusion in your meals.

Sources and Absorption of These Nutrients:

Familiarize yourself with the food sources rich in vitamin D, vitamin C, and iodine. Incorporate these nutrient-dense foods into your meal planning to ensure you are obtaining an adequate intake. Consider the absorption factors of these nutrients, such as pairing vitamin C-rich foods with iron-rich plant sources to enhance iron absorption.

Daily Recommended Intake of These Nutrients:

Be aware of the recommended daily intake of vitamin D, vitamin C, and iodine. Use this information as a guide when planning your meals to ensure you are meeting your nutrient needs. Keep in mind that individual requirements may vary based on factors such as age, sex, health conditions, and lifestyle.

Now, let's dive into some practical meal planning tips to help you optimize your nutrient intake:

Consider incorporating a variety of foods from different food groups to ensure a well-rounded nutrient profile. Include vitamin D, vitamin C, and iodine-rich foods in your meal plan to meet your specific nutrient needs.

Include Nutrient-Dense Foods: Fill your plate with a colorful array of fruits, vegetables, whole grains, lean proteins, and healthy fats. These foods provide a wealth of essential nutrients, including vitamin D, vitamin C, and iodine. Experiment with different recipes and cooking methods to keep your meals exciting and flavorful.

Focus on Natural Food Sources: Prioritize whole, unprocessed foods in your meal planning. Choose fresh fruits, vegetables, and seafood whenever possible to maximize your intake of these nutrients. Opt for minimally processed options to retain the highest nutrient content.

Balance Your Plate: Strive for a balanced meal by including a variety of food groups. Aim to fill half of your plate with colorful fruits and vegetables, one-quarter with lean proteins (including vitamin D-rich fish), and one-quarter with whole grains or other complex carbohydrates.

Snack Smartly: Incorporate nutrient-dense snacks between meals to further boost your intake of these essential nutrients. Opt for vitamin C-rich fruits, nuts and seeds, Greek yogurt, or seaweed snacks to satisfy cravings while providing valuable nutrients.

Stay Hydrated: Hydration is essential for nutrient absorption and overall well-being. Include water, herbal teas, and other hydrating beverages in your meal plan to support optimal nutrient utilization.

Remember, meal planning is a flexible and adaptable process. Adjust your plan based on seasonal availability of foods, individual preferences, and any specific dietary considerations you may have. Be open to experimenting with new recipes and flavors to keep your meals exciting and enjoyable.

Bon appétit!

Printed in Great Britain
by Amazon

28280935R00073